Juicing
4
A
Better
Life

Kevin D Passmore

Chapters

Chapter 1 Juicing & Who's This Book Is For

Juicing what is it? Regardless of what you call it, fast, cleanse or detox. What ever you want to call this, I want to make one thing clear, it is not a diet. What juicing is, and this book will allow you to do is

- Cleanse the body from all toxins
- Shrink Stomach to fill fuller faster
- Add Vitamin and Minerals back into the body

Now why is this book not a diet, is it because you wont lose weight? No, of course not you will loses weight while juicing, the longer you are juicing you will lose weight. The problem is you will be losing water weight, muscle and fat. So basically you will be losing everything, including the kitchen sink. The calorie restrictions are usually very strict, and you will not be getting all of the required nutrient from a normal diet. This book is set up using juicing as a starting point to begin the best possible you their can be. I know this is the beginning of the book but this is where it gets tricky. Their is no set plan for you and how you want to use Juicing. You will begin juicing for a minimum of 3 days, and recommend not juicing exclusively for more than 30 days. The tricky part is that I am not you, and none of us are the same. If your weight allows you to juice exclusively for more than 30 days ,and you are taking required supplements to stay healthy then by all means continue. If you cant make it exclusively on a juicing diet for 3 days, that's fine too, we will add in more food as we go. Their are no wrong answers to this, the goal is to make sure you are healthy, have energy and are losing weight properly. The eventual food choices for you after completing this book is to eat better and healthier food. Maintain a healthy life style using a variety of food that allows you the physical energy to live a long and healthy life. Now like I said earlier this is not a diet, even though I keep calling it a diet. I do that because I want to and Im writing the book, so I can. No I say this because Juicing would be considered a Fad diet. Their are a lot of fad diets that are effective and people maintain in a healthy manner. Some of those Fad diets will be discussed later on as options for expanded food choices. Some of those choices are the Paleo diet (Yes its a fad diet), Zone diet, South Beach Diet, and the Atkins Diet. The layout of this book will be similar to the Atkins Diet, we will have Phases. Phase I being the Juicing Phase, every phase will have a certain amount of time recommending you to be on it. When you move to the next phase you not only receive more food per meal but also more food options.

Chapter 2 A History of Juicing

The Dead Sea Scrolls have revealed that mashing pomegranate and figs for "profound strength and subtle form" was practiced from before 150 b.c. This is perhaps the first record of man's attempt to separate the vital juices from fruits and vegetables for their healing benefits.

Throughout the ages, herbalists and other health practitioners have grated or ground fresh herbs and soft fruits and pressed the juice along with the healing, active constituents from them. Dr. Max Gerson was the first to put forth the concept that diet could be used as cancer (and other disease) therapy, but it wasn't until the 1930s, when author and raw food proponent Dr. Norman Walker invented the first juicing machine, that juicing became widely available. 1954 was the year the first masticating juicer was invented, first named as the Champion Juicer. It was the best juicer at the time since it could juice almost every type of fruit and vegetable.

During the 1970s American fitness, nutrition and exercise expert, and motivational speaker Jack Lalanne began actively tackling the power of juicing and the health benefits from non-processed, natural foods. He introduced a line of juicers called "Jack Lalanne's Power Juice," which inspired Lalanne to make the famous quote, "That's the power of the juice!"

In 1993, the first twin gear juicer called The Green power Juicer was invented by a Korean man named Mr. Kim. The twin gear extraction process was based on the basic mortar and pestle concept which involves pressing the produce and getting most of the goodness of the fruits and vegetables. As a result, the live nutrients and enzymes are still intact which could have been destroyed and oxidized due to the high-speed rotating blades of the centrifugal juicer.

From 1990's onwards, juicing and juicers have become more popular and as a result more top rated juicers have been readily available on the market.

In 2000's up to present, several juicer reviews and articles have helped consumers in buying the ideal juicer, and experts are still doing a lot of research about juicing and its wonderful benefits. Efforts are still being made to further improve the juicers on the market.

Nowadays, people who want to embark on a healthy lifestyle will enjoy lots of juicer brands and configurations to choose from. It just means that we definitely have come a long way from the ancient era and the early 20th century yet still the methods of extracting juice are not so drastically different. And the first three juicers, The Norwalk, The Champion and The Green Power Juicer are actually still available on the market.

Chapter 3 Juicing & Diet Plan

As I stated earlier, you do not have to follow this time line that I am stating completely. Most importantly through this process is not only finding a healthy alternative to your current lifestyle. But also to develop food choices that are built on health, lifestyle and taste.
What do I mean by lifestyle choices?
Lifestyle choices will come into play when you start to take over the reigns more in the process of moving from this book into the real world where there are fast food options, pizza parties, soda and beer in the refrigerator. Here you are trying to develop a lifestyle where most of the time you are able to eat healthy and style delve into normal practices of guilt free indulgence without relapsing back into a state of mind where bad food choices remain a constant. Another example of lifestyle choices is that if you do not have time to eat six meals a day or have a schedule where you usually have to miss lunch then Breakfast, Lunch and Dinner is not a good idea for you. Maybe Intermediate Fasting is for you where you have a set time frame of 8 hours in a 24 hour day to eat all of your calorie for that day and consume no food or calories with the remaining 16 hour. Again I can not harp on this enough but this is your life, not mine, I don't know what is going on, I cant tell you what to do. I'm a book. No diet that you choose to do when transitioning from juicing to a more sustainable lifestyle is unhealthy. Every diet has its pros and cons, but not every diet works for everyone.
Some people can eat an entire pizza and lose weight. I hate those people, I for one have to monitor my calories, limit

cheat meals and maintain an active lifestyle to lose weight. I'm assuming most people here would be in the same boat. When I say no diet is unhealthy what I mean is that most diets are meant to be a sustainable lifestyle. So you need to enjoy the foods you are eating so you stay on it. If you enjoy Keto, or Paleo and the variety of food allowed makes you happy and is effective in keeping your weight off, then choose that diet. I for one love the Atkins Diet, a diet that is by everyone on the internet consider terrible for you. Why I mirror the Juicing Diet off of the Atkins Diet is because the Atkins Diet is the first diet that ever helped me lose weight. It was low in Calories which I needed to lose weight, It taught me a realistic portion size, and minimized Carbohydrates which makes my body gain weight.

So finally the Plan.

This will be broken down into different Phases

Phase I: Juicing Diet

Phase II: Vegan/ Vegetarian

Phase III: Calorie Maintenance

Phase IV: Freedom

Phase I Juicing Diet

Juicing 101

SUPPLIES

Go out and buy THREE 1-gallon jugs. You may want to grab one or two for times when juicing will be tougher/less convenient. Believe me, juicing is always easier when you have options on how to take it places.

Buy a Juicer online you can get one for 30-60 dollars that are relatively good and do not take up a lot of space.

Buy a stiff bristle brush for cleaning your juicer. I just went to the kitchen soap aisle at target and got one for like, $3. Believe me this makes life easier. Try to get thicker bristles as the smaller ones can catch in the juicing basket.

Your SHOPPING LIST for the grocery store
Note: you may have to adjust this. I buy kale in bags, for example, so I use 1/2 a bag for each recipe. Just try some different combos. Also, this should cost somewhere around $22. Use the Farmers Market when possible

Also note: This is configured to my tastes. I love the taste of this recipe, I know exactly what to buy, and I can make it in about 15 minutes. I don't mind drinking the same thing every day - you might. If you do, experiment with other recipes. Also, you can mess with this one and improve it. Don't like the tomato taste? Don't put em in! But replace it with, say, another cucumber. Or with bell peppers. Or with beets. Onion. Garlic. Etc.

-Grocery List
2lbs Carrots
1 whole bunch celery
2 Large Cucumbers
5-6 Roma Tomatoes
1 large yellow squash
4 Large Oranges
3 Large Lemons
2 thumb size pieces of whole ginger root (fresh)
1 Bag Spinach
1 Bag Kale

THE PREPARATION
Wash or soak your fruits and vegetables in water and baking soda or peel any of the veggies, peel the

oranges and lemons because their rinds make it bitter. I also cut the bottom off the celery to make it easier.

Put a plastic grocery bag in the pulp hopper. This aids in clean up! Thats it.

THE JUICING

Juice 1/2 of the Kale, 1/2 of the Spinach, you won't get much juice out of these but what you do get is packed with nutrients, 1.5 lbs Carrots all the rest of the items, juice the whole thing. This recipe follows standard sizes of items I can get at the market next to me, Celery, Tomatoes, and Ginger. Just put everything in whole. Have one of your gallon jugs by the juicer, as you'll need to empty the hopper into it periodically. Once you juice the ginger, you'll need to clean your juice-basket (since the ginger's so fibrous, it'll clog).

Clean the juicer filter basket with the brush you bought. Empty the pulp hopper. Put new grocery bag in hopper.

Juice the remaining ingredients. I juice the cucumbers last since they're so juicy they seem to rinse the juicer out - and bring the rest of the other juice with it.

Clean your juicer immediately afterwards so things do not dry in nooks and crannies that cant be seen or scrubbed. Never use the dishwasher to clean your juicer as it can warp the plastic.

Drink 44oz glasses a day and divide that up how ever you want, I only have two meals a day. 1 gallon will last 3 meals for me, or a day and a half for me. In the beginning if you start to feel weak, just drink more juice! You can't really drink too much of it. The sugar in it will make you feel better. A small 8oz glass will last you till your next meal usually. Though if you need to drink more, drink more!
After the first couple weeks, I would supplement the juice with just a bit of raw veggies to help fill you up. An example would be having a whole cucumber with a pinch of salt with dinner for example, or lightly steam some broccoli and put hot sauce on it. Find what works for you. Keep a bag of almonds or cashews around you. If you ever get hungry, I would count out 10-15 almonds, put away the bag and eat those. The fats in the almonds take away hunger pains.

Coffee is fine as long as its black. Water,Water, Water. You can not drink enough of it, whether it is water, lemon water, or tea drink it.

Things to expect during the first week You will fell a lot healthier after recovering from the initial mental fog. This fog should last between 2 and 5 days. Your skin should clear up, and you will have more energy (after the initial couple day shock).

Other Recipes for Variety are

-Drink Your Greens
2 Cups Spinach/ or 4-6 Kale Leaves
6 Celery Ribs
2 Cucumbers
½ Lemon
2 Medium Apples
1-2 In Ginger
1/4-1/2 Parsley Leaves

-Detoxifier
2-3 Medium Beets
6 Carrots
2 Medium Apples
½ Lemo
½ In Ginger

-The Vision
8 Large Carrots

2-3 Naval Oranges
1-2 In Ginger
1 In Turmer

-Sweet Carrot
10 Large Carrots
2 Medium Apples
¼ Cup Parsley (Optional)

-Greener Juice
4 leaves kale/ Celery

1 spear pineapple

1 small granny smith apple

2 stalks celery

-GRAPEFRUIT MINT JUICE
2 grapefruits peeled

1-2 inch ginger

2 sprigs mint

If you plan on making your own and I recommend
that you do try and make your own juices. Consider
this
have your greens and herbs washed and properly

stored in the refrigerator so they are ready to go. If

they're not, you may not be as motivated to juice.

•blend mostly vegetables with only a little fruit to make the juice not taste too bitter. I prefer to use one apple — peel, seeds, everything.

•if you want to juice low-liquid food, such as ginger or a clove of garlic, make sure you follow it with a high liquid vegetable such as carrot to flush it out of the juicer.

•clean your juicer as soon as possible after using it. I don't love cleaning my juicer, but I love it a whole lot less if it has been allowed to sit. Those fine vegetable fibers are way harder to get out of there once they've dried.

•the fresher the juice, the more nutrients it contains, but if you need to make your juice the night before, store it in a glass jar filled all the way up to the top so that there is a minimal amount of oxygen in contact with the juice. Cover and refrigerate.

These are the main fruits and vegetables used in Juicing and the reason why

Celery– low in calorie since it is mostly water. It is a low-glycemic food and a good source of dietary fiber, Vitamin A, Vitamin C, and Vitamin K.

Beets–contain nutrients that may help lower your

blood pressure, fight inflammation, and support detoxification.

Apples– "an apple a day keeps the doctor away" is a famous saying for good reason. Helps to fight inflammation and heart health.
Oranges– immune system booster since it is high in Vitamin C and low in calories.
Turmeric– anti-inflammatory and anti-oxidant properties
Ginger– aids in digestion and supports the immune system

How long you plan on Juicing is completely dependent on you. Try your best to stay on the Juicing phase for at least 3 days, if you have no side effects and it does not make it harder to live Id recommend Juicing for 2 weeks before moving on to Phase II. As I noted earlier, it is recommended to not Juice fore more than 30 days. If you have Juiced for less than 30 days and have lost 20 pounds, it is recommended that you transition to Phase II and add more whole food to your meals.

Phase II Vegan& Vegetarian

This is Phase II people, I hope that Juicing has benefited your overall life. Now it is time to add whole foods to your diet whether you have been eating whole vegetables and fruits during the Juicing period then you are right on track. If you want to continue to Juice for a certain Meal or with a meal that is completely up to you. If you want to transition over to whole foods completely also fine.

So Im sure a question you have is why Vegan/ Vegetarian? Its a simple reason which has nothing to do with converting you to a solely plant base diet. With Phase I you have the Detox or Cleanse where you are losing everything from your body. Phase II is a way to continue to have you eating similar things Fruits and Vegetables while being able to slowly... Slowly add calories to your diet to allow you to get a general base line of how many calories your body burns a day. During this phase expect your weight lose to not be as rapid as in the Juicing phase. Adding whole food back into your diet will also begin to stretch out you stomach after juicing which will make you feel full.

What is a Vegan Diet?

This is a plant based diet that refrains from consuming Meat, Dairy Product, and Egg. Im going to skip over the ethic portion of a Vegan diet. A vegan diet in a preliminary Clinical study found that it lowers the risk of type-2 diabetes, high blood pressure, obesity, and ischemic heart disease.

OK So What is Vegetarianism?

This is a Plant based diet that refrains from consuming Meat. Their are a few different types of Vegetarians that allow you to be closer to a vegan if you cut out Dairy products or eggs but it is your choice.

The reason you have the choice of Vegan or Vegetarian is because it is easier to get more protein as a vegetarian by consuming eggs and dairy. Again this is a personal choice, if you feel you are not lacking in Protein consumption start on a Vegan diet for a week to see how you would like to cycle in the new varieties of food to your daily life.

For phase II keep the meals simple, just like when Juicing find the foods that you like and want to eat regularly. This also means hopefully that you wont break the bank when it comes to grocery shopping. Buy Fruits and Vegetables that are in season, and do your best to buy natural food over frozen. Get to know your eating habits do you want 3 meals, 6 small meals, or are you going to be a grazer eating throughout the day. Allow yourself to eat til you are full but not stuffed.

Foods you are allowed to have
Vegetabes

Asparagus	Avacado
Beets	Bell Peppers
Broccoli	Brussels Sprouts
Cabbage	Carrots
Cauliflower	Celery
Corn	Cucumber
Eggplant	Garlic
Yams	Leeks
Mushrooms	Onion
Potatoes	Pumpkin
Radishes	Sprouts
Squash	Sugar Snap Peas
Sweet Potatoes	Tomatoes
Zuccini	

Leafy Greens

Arugula	Bok Choy
Kale	Lettuce
Romaine	Salad Mixes
Spinach	Spring Greens
Swiss Chard	Turnip Greens
Watercress	Wheatgrass

Fruit

Apples	Apricots
Bananas	Blackberries
Blueberries	Cherries
Grapefruit	Grapes
Kiwis	Lemon
Lime	Mangoes
Nectarines	Oranges
Peaches	Pears
Plums	Pomegranates
Raspberries	Strawberries
Watermelon	

Whole Grains

Amaranth	Barley
Rice (Brown, Wild)	Buckwheat
Bulgur	Cornflakes
Farro	Millet
Oats	Quinoa
Rye	Spelt
Whole Grain Pasta	

Legumes

Azuki Bean	Black Beans
Black Eyed Peas	Chickpeas
Edamame	Fava Beans
Green Beans	Kidney Beans
Lentils	Lima Beans
Mung Bean	Navy Bean
Pinto Bean	Red Beans
Snow Peas	Soy Beans
Split Peas	

Nuts

Almonds, Brazil Nuts, Cashews, Chestnuts, Hazelnuts, Macadamia Nuts, Pecans, Pine Nut, Pistachios, Walnuts

Seeds

Chia, Flax,Hemp, Pumpkin, Sesame, Sunflower
Seeds

Nuts & Butters
Almond, Cashew, Macadamia, Peanut Butter, Tahini

Dairy Substitute

Almond Milk	Cashew Milk
Coconut Milk	Coconut Yogurt
Hemp Milk	Oat Milk
Rice Milk	Soy Milk
Soy Yogurt	Temeh
Tofu	Vegan Cheese

For Vegetarians
Add to your Grocery List
Dairy, Cheese, and Eggs.

A Suggestion is to limit Cheese and Dairy intake due
to the fat content which in Phase I & II we are trying
to minimize.

Vegan Recipes

Breakfast
-Breakfast Tofu Scrambled Taco
Prep Time 5 Min/ Cook Time 10 Min

Ingredients

- 1 teaspoon olive oil
  1 red pepper, diced
  1 clove garlic, minced
  1 package super firm Tofu
  ¼ teaspoon ground turmeric
  ¼ teaspoon cumin
  ¼ teaspoon salt
  Freshly ground black pepper
  8 corn tortillas (can also use small whole grain tortillas)
  1 avocado, sliced
  ½ cup tomatoes
  ½ Cup Cheese

  -Breakfast Skillet
  Prep Time 5 Min/ Cook Time 15 Min
  1 Teaspoon Olive Oil
  1 Red Pepper Diced
  1 Cup Onion Diced
  4 Medium Potatoes
  2 Cup Spinach
  Lemon Juice
  Salt & Pepper to Taste

-Vegan Pancakes
Prep 10 Min/ Cook Time 10 Min

1 Cup Unbleached Flour
1 tbsp Cane Sugar
2 tsp Baking Powder
1/8 tsp Salt
1 Cup Soy/Almond Milk
1 tbsp Vinegar
2 tbsp Coconut Oil

-Protein Burrito
Prep 10 Min/ Cook Time 10 Min
½ Medium Red Onion
2 Garlic Cloves, Minced
12 oz Extra Firm Tofu
1 Tbsp Olive Oil
¼ tsp Turmeric
¼ tsp Cumin
½ Cup Black Beans
½ Avocado
½ Cup Salsa
Salt & Pepper to Taste
2 Large Whole Wheat Tortillas

-Broccoli & Quinoa Breakfast Patties
 Prep 5 Min/ Cook Time 20 Min
1 Cup Cooked Quinoa
2 Cups Low Sodium Vegetable Broth
1 cup Shredded Broccoli & Carrots
2 Flax Egg (1tbsp flax seed to 3 tbsp water makes 1 egg)
½ Cup Bread Crumb
2 garlic cloves minced
1 ½ tsp garlic powder
1 ½ tsp onion powder
3 tsp parsley
2 tbsp oil
Optional Salt, Pepper, Onion, Vegan Cheese

Vegan Lunch & Dinner

Simple to Complex Salads are delicious, get creative

-Banh Mi
Raw Veggies Shredded
3 ybsp Vegan White Wine
1 tsp Golden Caster Sugar
1 Long French Baguette
Hummus
Tempeh Finely Sliced
½ Small Pack Coriander Leaves
½ Small Pack Mint Leaves
1 tsp salt

Directions
Toss Vegetables in a bowl add vinegar sugar and salt let set to pickle. Heat Oven to 350 F, Cut Baguette into fours, then horizontally in half. Bake for 5 minutes until lightly brown. Spread hummus and tempeh slices and coat with pickled vegetables.

-Pasta Salad
Serves 4

8 oz Dried Pasta
15 oz Chickpeas
1 cup Broccoli, Shredded
½ Cup Carrot Sliced
½ Cup Red Onion, Sliced
¼ Cup Fresh Parsley
¼ Cup Olive Oil
¼ Cup Red Wine Vinegar
1 Clove Garlic Minced
1 tsp Dried Oregano
1 ½ Cup Cherry Tomatoes
Salt & Pepper to Taste

I know there are not a ton of option here but that is due to personal tastes as well as following a calorie restrictive diet 1600- 2000 calories you can create what ever you want. Use the internet to find recipes to diversify your options. These recipes emphasis more vegetables than whole grains and lentils. The goal at the start of phase II is to make sure you are getting enough protein, moderate carbohydrates and minimal fat in your diet. Fill up on vegetable over Rice, Beans and Lentils. Add Heavier carbohydrates like oats, Rice, Beans, and Lentils slowly to see how your body adapts to them. If you are anything like me carbohydrates are not friendly to losing weight. Follow Phase II for 1-4 weeks.

Phase III Calorie Maintenance

With Phase III you are doing exactly what it says, you have progressed slowly adding a variety of food. You know how much food you need to feel full, and do not over eat. You have developed good food habits in your everyday life and maintained these habits for over a month from phase I til now. Congratulation. If you have developed a love for Vegan or a vegetarian lifestyle, you are basically done. The goal for you is to enjoy life, enjoy food and maintain a healthy weight with your food choices. If you have not adopted a vegan or vegetarian lifestyle you are a blood thirsty murderer! Just kidding. Now you get to add Meat, Dairy, and Eggs to your diet. Basically here you get to go down a few different routes on how you change your diet. This is why the Vegan/ Vegetarian portion was so important to do. You allowed your body to learn how Carbohydrates are digested in your body. If Carbohydrates have no effect on your ability to lose weight your best bet for a future diet is the Paleolithic Diet. A Low Calorie Diet.

The Paleo Diet is a popular diet that covers a wide range of foods with the slogan, "Eat Meat and Vegetables, nuts and seeds, some fruit, little starch and no sugar".

If Carbohydrates cause a problem in your diet then you will like to look into the Atkins Diet. A low Carbohydrate Diet.

The Atkins Diet is a High Protein, moderate Fat and Low/ Moderate Carbohydrate diet.

The third category may be something that you find out after trying both of these diets first. This is the Pescetarianism where the only meat that you eat is seafood. Either this is an ethical reason or a diet heavy in meat is not gut healthy for you personally and eating seafood is lighter on the stomach.

Not to sound like a broken record but this decision is your choice. How these foods affect you, your lifestyle, and tastes are all up to you. What ever you do if you eat nothing but pizza and french fries remember that the only way any diet works is to be in a calorie deficit or maintenance.

Chapter 4 Fruits & Veggie Chart

for Vitamin and Minerals

Vitamin	What It Does	Its Found	
Biotin	Energy Storage	Avacado, Cauliflower, Eggs, Fruit, Liver, Pork, Salmon, Grain	
Folic Acid	• Prevention of birth defects • Protein metabolism • Red blood cell formation	• Asparagus • Avocado • Beans and peas • Enriched grain products (e.g., bread, cereal, pasta, rice) • Green leafy vegetables (e.g., spinach) • Orange juice	
Niacin	Cholesterol production • Conversion of food into energy • Digestion • Nervous system function	• Beans • Beef • Enriched grain products (e.g., bread, cereal, pasta, rice) • Nuts • Pork • Poultry • Seafood • Whole grains	
Pantothic Acid	Conversion of food into energy • Fat metabolism • Hormone production • Nervous system function • Red blood cell formation	• Avocados • Beans and peas • Broccoli • Eggs • Milk • Mushrooms • Poultry • Seafood • Sweet potatoes • Whole g	
Riboflavin	• Conversion of food into energy • Growth and development • Red blood cell	• Eggs • Enriched grain products (e.g., bread, cereal, pasta, rice) • Meats • Milk •	

	formation	Mushrooms • Poultry • Seafood (e.g., oysters) • Spinach	
Thiamin	• Conversion of food into energy • Nervous system function	• Beans and peas • Enriched grain products (e.g., bread, cereal, pasta, rice) • Nuts • Pork • Sunflower seeds • Whole grains	
Vitamin A	Growth and development • Immune function • Reproduction • Red blood cell formation • Skin and bone formation • Vision	Cantaloupe • Carrots • Dairy products • Eggs • Fortified cereals • Green leafy vegetables (e.g., spinach and broccoli) • Pumpkin • Red peppers • Sweet potatoes	
Vitamin B 6	Immune function • Nervous system function • Protein, carbohydrate, and fat metabolism • Red blood cell formation	• Chickpeas • Fruits (other than citrus) • Potatoes • Salmon • Tuna	
Vitamin B12	• Conversion of food into energy • Nervous system function • Red blood cell formation	• Dairy products • Eggs • Fortified cereals • Meats • Poultry • Seafood (e.g., clams, trout, salmon, haddock, tuna	
Vitamin C	• Antioxidant • Collagen and connective tissue formation • Immune function • Wound healing	Broccoli • Brussels sprouts • Cantaloupe • Citrus fruits and juices (e.g., oranges and	

		grapefruit) • Kiwifruit • Peppers • Strawberries • Tomatoes and tomato juice	
Vitamin D	• Blood pressure regulation • Bone growth • Calcium balance • Hormone production • Immune function • Nervous system function	• Eggs • Fish (e.g., herring, mackerel, salmon, trout, and tuna) • Fish liver oil • Fortified cereals • Fortified dairy products • Fortified margarine • Fortified orange juice • Fortified soy beverages (soymilk)	
Vitamin E	• Antioxidant • Formation of blood vessels • Immune function	• Fortified cereals and juices • Green vegetables (e.g., spinach and broccoli) • Nuts and seeds • Peanuts and peanut butter • Vegetable oils	

Mineral	What It Does	Its Found	Daily Value
Calcium	• Blood clotting • Bone and teeth formation • Constriction and relaxation of blood vessels • Hormone secretion • Muscle contraction • Nervous system function	• Almond, rice, coconut, and hemp milks • Canned seafood with bones (e.g., salmon and sardines) • Dairy products • Fortified cereals and juices • Fortified soy beverages	1000 mg

Chloride	• Acid-base balance • Conversion of food into energy • Digestion • Fluid balance • Nervous system function	(soymilk) • Green vegetables (e.g., spinach, kale, broccoli, turnip greens) • Tofu (made with calcium sulfate)	
Chloride	• Acid-base balance • Conversion of food into energy • Digestion • Fluid balance • Nervous system function	• Celery • Lettuce • Olives • Rye • Salt substitutes • Seaweeds (e.g., dulse and kelp) • Table salt and sea salt • Tomatoes	3400 mg
Chromium	• Insulin function • Protein, carbohydrate, and fat metabolism	• Broccoli • Fruits (e.g., apple and banana) • Grape and orange juice • Meats • Spices (e.g., garlic and basil) • Turkey • Whole grains	120 mcg
Copper	• Antioxidant • Bone formation • Collagen and connective tissue formation • Energy production • Iron metabolism • Nervous system function	• Chocolate and cocoa • Crustaceans and shellfish • Lentils • Nuts and seeds • Organ meats (e.g., liver) • Whole grains	2 mg
Iodine	• Growth and development • Metabolism • Reproduction • Thyroid hormone production	• Breads and cereals • Dairy products • Iodized salt • Potatoes • Seafood • Seaweed • Turkey	150 mg
Iron	• Energy production • Growth and development • Immune function • Red blood cell	• Beans and peas • Dark green vegetables • Meats • Poultry • Prunes and prune juice • Raisins •	18 mg

	formation • Reproduction • Wound healing	Seafood • Whole grain, enriched, and fortified cereals and breads	
Magnesium	• Blood pressure regulation • Blood sugar regulation • Bone formation • Energy production • Hormone secretion • Immune function • Muscle contraction • Nervous system function • Normal heart rhythm • Protein formation	• Avocados • Bananas • Beans and peas • Dairy products • Green leafy vegetables (e.g., spinach) • Nuts and pumpkin seeds • Potatoes • Raisins • Wheat bran • Whole grains	400 mg
Manganese	• Carbohydrate, protein, and cholesterol metabolism • Cartilage and bone formation • Wound healing	• Beans • Nuts • Pineapple • Spinach • Sweet potato • Whole grains	2 mg
Molybdenum	• Enzyme production	• Beans and peas • Nuts • Whole grains	75 mcg
Phosphorus	• Acid-base balance • Bone formation • Energy production and storage • Hormone activation	• Beans and peas • Dairy products • Meats • Nuts and seeds • Poultry • Seafood • Whole grain, enriched, and fortified cereals and breads	1000 mg
Potassium	• Blood pressure regulation • Carbohydrate metabolism • Fluid balance • Growth	• Bananas • Beet greens • Juices (e.g., carrot, pomegranate, prune, orange,	3500 mg

	and development • Heart function • Muscle contraction • Nervous system function • Protein formation	and tomato) • Milk • Oranges and orange juice • Potatoes and sweet potatoes • Prunes and prune juice • Spinach • Tomatoes and tomato products • White beans • Yogurt	
Selenium	• Antioxidant • Immune function • Reproduction • Thyroid function	• Eggs • Enriched pasta and rice • Meats • Nuts (e.g., Brazil nuts) and seeds • Poultry • Seafood • Whole grains	70 mcg
Sodium	• Acid-base balance • Blood pressure regulation • Fluid balance • Muscle contraction • Nervous system function	Breads and rolls • Cheese (natural and processed) • Cold cuts and cured meats (e.g., deli or packaged ham or turkey) • Mixed meat dishes (e.g., beef stew, chili, and meat loaf) • Mixed pasta dishes (e.g., lasagna, pasta salad, and spaghetti with meat sauce) • Pizza • Poultry (fresh and processed) • Sandwiches (e.g., hamburgers, hot dogs, and submarine sandwiches) • Savory snacks (e.g., chips, crackers, popcorn,	2400 mg

| | | and pretzels) • Soups • Table salt | |
| Zinc | • Growth and development • Immune function • Nervous system function • Protein formation • Reproduction • Taste and smell • Wound healing | • Beans and peas • Beef • Dairy products • Fortified cereals • Nuts • Poultry • Seafood (e.g., clams, crabs, lobsters, oysters) • Whole grains | 15 mg |

Chapter 5 Herbs & Spices for Ailments

Garlic	Antioxidant, lowers cholesterol and blood pressure, raises HDL cholesterol, anti-inflammatory, prevents cerebral aging, anti-clotting, boosts immunity
Ginger	Antioxidant, improves osteoarthritis of the knee, anti-emetic, anti-inflammatory, boosts immunity, antimicrobial
Lemon Grass	Antioxidant, anti-cancer properties, anti-inflammatory
Cilantro	Antioxidant, digestive aid
Chili	Antioxidant, enhances metabolic effects in weight management
Basil	Antioxidant, inhibits lipid peroxidation, decreases inflammation
Dill	Antioxidant, antimicrobial
Parsley	Antioxidant, antimicrobial
Oregano	Antioxidant, antimicrobial
Marjoram	Antioxidant, antimicrobial
Thyme	Antioxidant, inhibits bone

	resorption
Rosemary	Antioxidant, inhibits bone resorption, anti-carcinogen, anti-inflammatory
Cinnamon	Lower Blood Sugar
Sage	Improve Memory
Peppermint	Reduces Nausea
Turmeric	Anti Inflammatory
Fenugreek	Controls Blood Sugar

Teas

Chamomile	Sleep Aid
Peppermint	Improves Digestion
Ginger	Fights Inflammation
Hibiscus	Lowers Blood Pressure
Echinacea	Fights Common Cold
Rooibos	Lowers Blood Pressure
Sage	Fights Alzheimers
Lemon Balm	Fights Heart Disease
Rose Hip	Anti Inflammation, High Vitamin C
Passion Flower	Reduce Anxiety, Improve Sleep

Chapter 6 Planning Your Future Health

What ever your future hold with your food remember these simple steps to get back on track.

1.Start your Diet off Right

If you've been restricting food but not counting calories—this is more common than you might think—then our first recommendation is to perform an honest audit of your current intake. Spend the next three days tracking your daily macronutrients—that is, number of grams of protein, carbs, and fats—and establish a caloric baseline. You can use the old pen-and-paper method, or utilize any of the popular nutrition-tracking apps like MyMacros+ or MyFitnessPal. More importantly, don't change yet. Do your best to be as honest as possible about what and how much you truly eat. Once you've got that number, it's time to tweak it. Most people will find that dieting on a bodyweight multiplier of 12 for total calories is a good starting point. In other words, take your body weight in pounds and multiply that by 12 to determine your total intake for the day. So if you weigh 150 pounds, then 1,800 calories per day will be your goal for fat loss. If you started far lower than body weight-times-12 in the past, that could be precisely what led you down the road to adaptation.

2.Add Calories Back In Slowly

The lower your calories the crummier you feel, and the more aggressive you may want to be with your increase in calories. Otherwise slow and steady is best, increase 2-10 percent per week.

3. Find Small Changes To Boost Adherence

Consider shaking up your diet by improving the target macro nutrient numbers. It is a constant battle to track your calorie intake depending on your calorie output. Example if you want to increase your calorie intake consider incorporating exercises to stay in a maintenance phase.